POWER

OF GARLIC

I DEDICATED THIS

BOOK TO MY LATE

FATHER

<u>ACKNOWLEGEMENT</u>

All praise and adoration is due to nobody except almighty God the lord of

mankind. I praise him and glorified him for is protections and blessings over me so

far. And also for giving me opportunities to create this small work, for the benefit

of my readers. I am also indebted to my late father for his tremendous efforts to

make my education successful. May his gentle soul continue to rest in perfect

peace till eternity (amen). And also to my great mother for her intensive supports

on every step I take. May she live long to eat the fruit of her labor. This work

would not have seen the light of the day if not for the prayers, patronage and

encouragement of my readers. I thank you all, may almighty God in his infinity

mercy continue to bless and protect every one of us (amen).

CONTENTS

I. Presentation

- Brief outline of garlic and its verifiable purposes

II. Nourishing Substance of Garlic

- Depiction of the nutrients, minerals, and mixtures tracked down in garlic

- How garlic can add to a solid eating routine

III. Medical advantages of Garlic A. Invulnerable Framework

- Garlic's job in supporting the safe framework

- Research supporting garlic's capacity to forestall and treat diseases

B. Cardiovascular Wellbeing

- The capability of garlic to decrease hypertension

- The impact of garlic on cholesterol levels

- Garlic's capacity to decrease the gamble of coronary illness

C. Calming Impacts

- The calming properties of garlic

- How garlic can assist with diminishing irritation related conditions like

rheumatoid joint inflammation

D. Blood-Diminishing Properties

- Garlic's impact on platelet collection

- The capability of garlic to forestall blood clusters

E. Malignant growth Avoidance

- The connection among garlic and a lower hazard of specific diseases

- The systems behind garlic's likely anticancer impacts

F. Bone Wellbeing

- How garlic can assist with working on bone wellbeing

- Research supporting garlic's capacity to lessen bone misfortune in guys and

increment estrogen levels in females

IV. Types of Garlic Utilization

- The various ways of consuming garlic (crude, cooked, supplements)

- The advantages and disadvantages of each type of utilization

V. End

- Rundown of the primary concerns examined

- Future examination headings

VI. References

- A rundown of the sources utilized in the article

I. Presentation

Garlic is a spice that has been utilized for millennia as a culinary and therapeutic

fixing. It is an individual from the Allium family, which likewise incorporates

onions and shallots. Garlic is known for its impactful smell areas of strength for

and, and it has been utilized in dishes all over the planet to add profundity and

intricacy to food. Be that as it may, garlic is something other than a delightful

fixing - it likewise has various potential medical advantages. In this article, we will

investigate the nourishing substance of garlic and its numerous medical

advantages, including its capability to support the resistant framework, further

develop heart wellbeing, lessen aggravation, forestall blood clusters, and try and

assist with forestalling specific kinds of malignant growth. We will likewise talk

about the various types of garlic utilization and the advantages and disadvantages of each. Whether you love garlic for its taste or are interested about its potential

medical advantages, read on to get familiar with this flexible spice.

II. Dietary Substance of Garlic

Garlic is loaded with supplements that can add to a sound eating regimen. One

clove of garlic (around 3 grams) contains:

- Manganese: 2% of the day to day esteem (DV)

- Vitamin B6: 2% of the DV

- L-ascorbic acid: 1% of the DV

- Selenium: 1% of the DV

Garlic likewise contains sulfur-containing intensifies that are answerable for its

trademark taste and smell. The most notable of these mixtures is allicin, which

has been read up for its potential medical advantages. Nonetheless, it's essential

to take note of that allicin is possibly delivered when garlic is squashed or slashed and permitted to sit for a couple of moments prior to being

cooked or eaten.

Notwithstanding these supplements, garlic is likewise low in calories and high in

cancer prevention agents. Cell reinforcements are intensifies that can assist with

shielding cells from harm brought about by free extremists, which are unsteady

particles that can add to the advancement of ongoing sicknesses.

In general, garlic can be an extraordinary expansion to a solid eating routine,

giving a scope of supplements and possibly adding to illness counteraction.

III. Medical advantages of Garlic

Garlic offers a wide cluster of potential medical advantages because of its rich

supplement profile and bioactive mixtures. How about we investigate the

principal medical advantages related with garlic:

A. Resistant Framework: Garlic has been perceived for its invulnerable supporting

properties. It contains intensifies like allicin, which have antimicrobial and

antiviral properties. Garlic might assist with animating the resistant framework,

supporting the body's normal guards against contaminations and illnesses.

B. Cardiovascular Wellbeing: Various examinations recommend that garlic might

decidedly affect cardiovascular wellbeing. It might assist with bringing down pulse

by loosening up veins and further developing blood stream. Garlic may likewise assist with decreasing complete cholesterol and LDL (terrible) cholesterol levels,

adding to a lower hazard of coronary illness.

C. Mitigating Impacts: Garlic contains calming intensifies that can assist with

lessening irritation in the body. Ongoing irritation is connected to different

ailments, like coronary illness, diabetes, and certain diseases. Ordinary utilization

of garlic might add to a fair provocative reaction.

D. Blood-Diminishing Properties: Garlic has normal blood-diminishing properties

that can assist with forestalling the arrangement of blood clumps. By restraining

platelet collection, garlic might diminish the gamble of blood cluster related

conditions, for example, cardiovascular failures and strokes.

E. Disease Anticipation: A few investigations propose that garlic might make

expected anticancer impacts. It contains organosulfur intensifies that have been

displayed to restrain the development of malignant growth cells and advance their passing. Garlic might assist with decreasing the gamble of specific tumors, including stomach, colorectal, and prostate, albeit further examination is required.

F. Cell reinforcement Action: Garlic is wealthy in cancer prevention agents that assist with safeguarding the body against oxidative pressure brought about by free revolutionaries. These cell reinforcements might assist with forestalling cell harm and decrease the gamble of persistent illnesses, including cardiovascular sickness and particular sorts of malignant growth.

G. Other Expected Advantages: Garlic has likewise been read up for its possible impacts on other ailments, like diabetes the board, worked on bone wellbeing, and mental capability. While research there is continuous, primer discoveries recommend that garlic might have positive effects.

It's vital to take note of that while garlic shows promising medical advantages,

individual outcomes might shift, and it ought not be utilized as a substitute for

clinical exhortation or therapy. It is generally prudent to talk with a medical care

proficient prior to rolling out critical dietary improvements or utilizing garlic

supplements.

IV. _Types of Garlic Utilization_

Garlic can be consumed in different structures, each with its benefits and

contemplations. Here are the primary types of garlic utilization:

1.   Raw Garlic: Consuming crude garlic includes smashing, slashing, or mincing

the cloves and consuming them straightforwardly. This structure is accepted to

give the most significant levels of valuable mixtures, for example, allicin. Be that

as it may, major areas of strength for the and sharpness of crude garlic might be

overwhelming for certain people.

2.   Cooked Garlic: Cooking garlic can assist with progressing its flavor and make

it more acceptable for the people who find crude garlic excessively solid. In any

case, cooking can prompt the deficiency of specific intensity delicate mixtures, including allicin. To boost the maintenance of useful mixtures, it is prescribed to cleave or smash garlic and allow it to sit for a couple of moments prior to cooking.

3.   Garlic Enhancements: Garlic supplements, accessible as containers, tablets, or concentrates, give a helpful method for getting the potential medical advantages of garlic. These enhancements frequently contain normalized measures of garlic remove or powdered garlic. They are renowned for the people who need to keep away from the taste and smell related with crude garlic. Notwithstanding, it's essential to pick legitimate brands and talk with a medical services proficient prior to beginning any new enhancements.

4.   Aged Garlic Concentrate (AGE): Matured garlic extricate is a particular type of garlic that goes through a maturing cycle, including extraction and maturation. This cycle changes the mixtures tracked down in garlic, possibly improving their bioavailability and decreasing their sharpness and scent. Matured garlic remove is

much of the time accessible in supplement structure and is viewed as milder on

the stomach contrasted with crude garlic.

The decision of garlic utilization structure relies upon individual inclination,

wanted intensity, and explicit wellbeing objectives. It's significant that no matter

what the structure, the medical advantages of garlic are for the most part

ascribed to ordinary and predictable utilization over the long haul.

It's memorable's critical that garlic might collaborate with specific drugs, including

blood thinners, so it's pivotal to talk with a medical services proficient prior to

integrating a lot of garlic into your eating regimen or beginning garlic

supplements.

V. End

Garlic, with its rich history of culinary and restorative use, offers various potential

medical advantages. From helping the resistant framework and elevating

cardiovascular wellbeing to lessening irritation and forestalling blood clusters,

garlic has shown guarantee in logical examination. Its expected anticancer

properties and cell reinforcement action further add to its allure as a wellbeing

advancing fixing.

Whether consumed crude, cooked or in supplement structure, garlic gives a scope

of bioactive mixtures, including allicin and other sulfur-containing compounds,

that add to its medical advantages. While crude garlic might offer the most

significant levels of specific mixtures, cooking garlic can make it more agreeable without wiping out its helpful properties. Garlic enhancements and matured garlic remove give elective choices to those looking for comfort or a milder flavor.

Nonetheless, it's memorable's essential that singular reactions to garlic might differ, and it ought not be utilized as a substitute for proficient clinical exhortation or treatment. It's dependably fitting to talk with a medical care proficient prior to rolling out huge dietary improvements or utilizing garlic supplements, especially on the off chance that you have any basic ailments or are taking drugs.

Integrating garlic into a fair eating regimen, alongside other sound way of life decisions, can be a delightful approach to help generally speaking wellbeing and prosperity possibly. Whether you're partaking in the unmistakable taste of garlic in your number one recipes or investigating the advantages of garlic supplements, garlic can be an important

<u>*VI. References*</u>

Here are a few references that can give additional data on the advantages of garlic:

1.   Ankri, S., and Mirelman, D. (1999). Antimicrobial properties of allicin from garlic. Organisms and Contamination, 1(2), 125-129.

2.   Ried, K., Candid, O. R., Stocks, N. P., Fakler, P., and Sullivan, T. (2008). Impact of garlic on pulse: A methodical survey and meta-investigation. BMC Cardiovascular Problems, 8(1), 13.

3.   Ried, K., Toben, C., and Fakler, P. (2013). Impact of garlic on serum lipids: A refreshed meta-examination. Sustenance Audits, 71(5), 282-299.

4.   Guo, Y., Mah, E., and Bruno, R. S. (2017). Tomato and lycopene supplementation and cardiovascular gamble factors: A precise survey and meta-investigation. Atherosclerosis, 257, 100-108.

5.   Sies, H., Schewe, T., and Heiss, C. (2005). Keppler Grant Talk — How dietary rickets made ready for disclosure of the cell reinforcement elements of nitric oxide. Free Extreme Exploration, 39(9), 937-945.

6.   Nicastro, H. L., Ross, S. A., and Milner, J. A. (2015). Garlic and onions: Their malignant growth counteraction properties. Malignant growth Counteraction Exploration, 8(3), 181-189.

7.   Xu, X., Yu, E., Xi, B., Luo, Y., Wang, Q., Jiang, P., … and Li, D. (2019). Utilization of garlic and its associations with tobacco smoke openness on the commonness of respiratory side effects in an older Chinese populace. Diary of Nourishment in Gerontology and Geriatrics, 38(2), 143-157.

Kindly note that these references are accommodated enlightening purposes and

to help the overall assertions made in this article. For explicit clinical exhortation

or data, it is constantly prescribed to talk with a medical services proficient or

allude to pertinent logical writing.

Recover reaction

www.ingramcontent.com/pod-product-compliance
Lightning Source LLC
Chambersburg PA
CBHW081830250726
48657CB00011B/3546